Covid 19 pandemic

A professional research guide on covid 19 syrup potential solution to covid19 pandemic

Dr Joe smith

Contents

chapter1

introduction to covid19 syrup

The COVID-19 pandemic has affected the entire world since it first emerged in December 2019 in Wuhan, China. This highly infectious disease, caused by the SARS-CoV-2 virus, has spread rapidly and has resulted in millions of cases and hundreds of thousands of deaths across the globe. As medical professionals and researchers have worked tirelessly to develop effective treatments, a new potential solution has emerged - COVID-19 syrup. COVID-19 syrup, also known as COVID syrup, is a herbal treatment that claims to boost the immune system and provide relief from the symptoms of COVID-19. It has gained popularity in recent months as people search for alternative treatments for this highly contagious and deadly virus. What is COVID-19 Syrup? COVID-19 syrup is a mixture of various herbs and natural ingredients that are believed to have anti-viral and immune-boosting properties. These ingredients may include ginger, turmeric, black pepper, honey, and various other herbs and spices. The syrup is commonly consumed orally, with a recommended dosage of one to two tablespoons daily. The makers of COVID-19 syrup claim that it can help prevent and treat COVID-19 infections by boosting the body's immune system and reducing the severity of symptoms. However, there is limited scientific evidence to support these claims, and the effectiveness of the syrup is still under debate. Development of COVID-19 Syrup The development of COVID-19 syrup can be attributed to the widespread use of herbal remedies in traditional medicine. With the rise in cases of COVID-19, many herbal practitioners have started promoting this syrup as a potential treatment for the virus. In countries like India, where traditional medicine has a strong cultural influence, herbal remedies have been widely used to treat various ailments for centuries. Therefore, it was not surprising when various Ayurvedic companies in India started promoting COVID-19 syrup as a way to combat the virus. The government of India, in an effort to find a suitable treatment for COVID-19, even urged the Indian

Council of Medical Research (ICMR) to conduct a study on the potential benefits of these herbal remedies. As a result, several trials and studies are currently underway to determine the effectiveness of COVID-19 syrup in treating COVID-19. Potential Benefits of COVID-19 Syrup? Supporters of COVID-19 syrup claim that it has many potential benefits, including boosting the immune system and reducing the severity of COVID-19 symptoms. The various ingredients in the syrup are believed to have anti-inflammatory and anti-viral properties, which may help in fighting the virus and supporting the body's defenses. Additionally, proponents of the syrup argue that it is a natural and holistic approach to treating COVID-19, which may be preferred by those who are hesitant to use Western medicines or are looking for alternative treatments. It is also more affordable compared to traditional medications, making it an attractive option for those who cannot afford expensive treatments. However, there is limited scientific evidence to support these claims. While some studies have shown potential anti-viral properties of some of the ingredients in COVID-19 syrup, there is no conclusive evidence that it can treat or prevent COVID-19. Controversies Surrounding COVID-19 Syrup Like any new treatment, COVID-19 syrup has faced its fair share of controversies. One of the major concerns is the lack of scientific evidence to support its claims. While many people believe in the benefits of herbal remedies, there is a need for robust scientific studies to verify their effectiveness. Moreover, there have been reports of fake COVID-19 syrups being sold in the market, which can be potentially harmful to people's health. The lack of proper regulation and quality control in the production of these syrups has raised concerns among health experts and government bodies. Another major concern is the potential for the syrup to be misused as a replacement for established Western medicines. COVID-19 is a highly contagious and deadly virus, and relying solely on unproven herbal remedies can be dangerous and even fatal. Do We Need More Research? In light of the controversies surrounding COVID-19 syrup, there is a growing need for more research and studies to be conducted to determine its effectiveness. The ICMR has already initiated trials, and other organizations and researchers are also working to gather more data on the potential benefits of the syrup. In addition to its possible effects on COVID-19, it is essential to study the safety and side effects of consuming large quantities of these herbs and spices. Some of these ingredients may have interactions with other medications and could potentially cause harm to people with certain medical conditions. Final Thoughts In conclusion, COVID-19 syrup is a herbal remedy that has gained popularity as a potential treatment for COVID-19. While its supporters claim numerous benefits, there is limited scientific evidence to support its effectiveness. There are also concerns about the proper regulation and misuse of these syrups. As the world continues to battle the COVID-19 pandemic, it is important to rely on reliable and scientifically proven treatments. While herbal remedies may provide some relief and support, they should not be used as a replacement for established medical treatments. More research and studies are needed to fully understand the potential benefits and risks of COVID-19 syrup. In the meantime, it is crucial to follow proper health guidelines and rely on approved treatments to combat the virus.

best cough syrup for covid19 patient

A cough is a natural reflex that helps to clear the airways of irritants, mucus, and other foreign substances. However, with COVID-19, coughing can become severe and persistent, leading to complications such as difficulty in breathing and increased risk of spreading the virus to others. Therefore, it is essential to find a cough syrup that can help relieve symptoms and suppress the urge to cough in COVID-19 patients. When it comes to selecting the best cough syrup for COVID-19 patients, there are several factors that one needs to consider. These include the ingredients, effectiveness, side effects, and overall safety of the cough syrup. Here, we will discuss some of the top cough syrups that have been recommended by medical professionals for the treatment of COVID-19 patients.

1.   Dextromethorphan-based Cough Syrups Dextromethorphan is an active ingredient, known for its cough-suppressing properties. It is commonly used in over-the-counter cough syrups and is a recommended option for COVID-19 patients. Dextromethorphan works by suppressing the cough reflex at the brainstem, reducing the urge to cough. This not only provides relief to the patient but also helps in preventing the spread of the virus to others. Some

of the popular cough syrups that contain dextromethorphan include Robitussin, Mucinex DM, and Delsym. These syrups come in different formulations and flavors, making them easy to consume for patients. However, it is essential to note that dextromethorphan can cause side effects such as dizziness, drowsiness, and dry mouth. Therefore, it is crucial to follow the recommended dosage and consult with a medical professional before taking any of these cough syrups. 2. Guaifenesin-based Cough Syrups Guaifenesin is another active ingredient found in cough syrups that can help COVID-19 patients. It is an expectorant that works by thinning and loosening mucus in the airways, making it easier to cough up. This property is highly beneficial for patients with COVID-19 as it can help in keeping the airways clear and reducing the severity of coughing. Popular cough syrups that contain guaifenesin include Robitussin Mucus + Chest Congestion, Mucinex, and Cheracol. These syrups are known for providing fast and effective relief to patients, especially those with productive coughs. However, some side effects of guaifenesin-based cough syrups may include nausea, vomiting, and headaches. Therefore, it is essential to consult with a doctor before consuming these syrups, especially if you have underlying health conditions.

3. Honey-based Cough Syrups Honey has been used as a natural remedy for coughs and colds for centuries. It is

known for its antibacterial and anti-inflammatory properties, making it an excellent option for COVID-19 patients. Honey-based cough syrups help in soothing the throat, reducing coughing, and providing relief from symptoms associated with the virus. One of the most popular honey-based cough syrups is Buckleys Mixture, which contains a combination of honey, menthol, camphor, and lemon. It is known for its soothing and healing effects on the respiratory system. However, it is important to note that honey-based cough syrups are not recommended for children under the age of one due to the risk of infant botulism. 4. Codeine-based Cough Syrups Codeine is an opioid drug that is often used in combination with other active ingredients in cough syrups. It is known for its pain-relieving and cough-suppressing properties. Codeine-based cough syrups are highly effective in providing relief to patients with severe and persistent coughs, especially those caused by COVID-19. Popular codeine-based cough syrups include Cheratussin, Robitussin AC, and Tuzistra XR. However, it is important to note that codeine is a controlled substance and can cause side effects such as dizziness, drowsiness, and constipation. Therefore, it is essential to follow the recommended dosage and consult with a doctor before taking any of these cough syrups. 5. Bromhexine-based Cough Syrups Bromhexine is an active ingredient found in cough syrups that works by thinning and loosening mucus in the lungs, making it easier to cough up. It is also known for its anti-inflammatory and antioxidant properties, which can be beneficial for COVID-19 patients. Bromhexine-based cough syrups are commonly used to treat productive coughs and provide relief to patients experiencing chest congestion. Popular cough syrups that contain bromhexine include Bisolvon, Mucolyxir, and Robitussin Chesty Cough. These syrups are known for their effectiveness in reducing coughing and providing relief from other symptoms associated with COVID-19. However, bromhexine can cause side effects such as nausea, stomach discomfort, and skin rashes in some patients. Therefore, it is essential to consult with a doctor before taking any of these cough syrups.

chapter2

how to treat covid cough

1. Isolate Yourself If you have developed a cough, it is crucial to isolate yourself immediately. This means staying at home and avoiding contact with others to prevent the spread of the virus. If you live with other people, it is essential to wear a face mask to avoid infecting them. Do not share any personal items such as cups, plates, or utensils with others and try to stay in a separate room to minimize contact with others. 2. Stay Hydrated Coughing can be very dehydrating, so it is essential to drink plenty of fluids to keep your body hydrated. Water is the best option, but

you can also drink herbal tea, clear soups, and fruit juices. Avoid caffeinated and carbonated drinks, as they can worsen your cough. Staying hydrated helps in thinning the mucus in your airways, making it easier to expel and reducing the frequency of your coughing. 3. Use a Humidifier or Steam A dry cough can be very uncomfortable and often leads to more severe coughing fits. To ease your cough, try using a humidifier or inhaling steam. A humidifier adds moisture to the air, which can soothe your throat and reduce coughing. You can also place a damp towel over your head and breathe in steam from a pot of boiling water. Adding a few drops of essential oils like eucalyptus or peppermint can also help relieve congestion and soothe your cough. 4. Gargle with Salt Water Gargling with warm salt water can help to reduce the pain and irritation caused by a cough. Saltwater gargles also help to clear mucus from the back of your throat, reducing coughing. Mix half a teaspoon of salt in a glass of warm water and gargle for 30 seconds. Repeat several times a day for best results. 5. Use Over-the-Counter Medications There are several over-the-counter medications that can help relieve a Covid cough. Cough syrups containing expectorants, like guaifenesin, can help thin and loosen mucus, making it easier to cough up. Cough suppressants, such as dextromethorphan, can help reduce the frequency of your coughing.

However, it is essential to consult with a doctor or pharmacist before taking any medications to ensure they do not interact with any other medications you may be taking. 6. Try Natural Remedies Many natural remedies can help ease a Covid cough. These include ginger, honey, and turmeric. Ginger has anti-inflammatory properties and can help relieve sore throat and coughing. Honey is a natural cough suppressant and can also soothe a sore throat. Turmeric has antibacterial and anti-inflammatory properties that can help improve lung health and reduce a cough. You can add these ingredients to tea or hot water for maximum benefits. 7. Practice Breathing Techniques Deep breathing and relaxation techniques can help relieve a

Covid cough. Breathing deeply can calm your body and may help control a coughing fit. You can try simple breathing exercises, such as inhaling slowly through your nose and exhaling through your mouth. Practicing meditation or yoga can also help relax your body and reduce the frequency of your coughing. 8. Avoid Irritants Avoid exposure to any irritants that may trigger your cough, such as smoke, dust, or pollution. These irritants can aggravate your cough and make it harder to control. If you are a smoker, it is crucial to quit smoking immediately to prevent further damage to your lungs and respiratory system. 9. Get Plenty of Rest Resting is essential to help your body fight off the virus and recover.

Avoid any strenuous activities that may worsen your cough. Adequate rest will also help boost your immune system and reduce the severity of your symptoms. It is recommended to get at least 8 hours of sleep each night to allow your body to heal and recover. 10. Seek Medical Attention If your cough persists for more than a week or if you experience difficulty breathing, chest pain, or other severe symptoms, it is essential to seek medical attention immediately. These could be signs of a more severe infection, and a doctor will be able to provide you with the appropriate treatment.

chapter3

delsym for covid cough

Delsym, a commonly used cough suppressant and expectorant, has emerged as a potential treatment for the persistent cough associated with COVID-19. As the world continues to battle the deadly pandemic caused by the novel coronavirus, studies have shown that many patients experience a lingering cough even after the infection has cleared. This post-COVID cough can be severe, lasting for weeks or even months, causing discomfort and hindering the recovery process for many individuals. In this article, we will explore the effectiveness of Delsym in managing the COVID cough and its potential role in treating this lingering symptom. Delsym, also known by its generic name dextromethorphan, is a cough suppressant that works by suppressing the cough reflex in the brain. It is commonly used to relieve coughs caused by the common cold, flu, and other respiratory infections. The medication is available in various forms, including tablets, liquid, and lozenges. However, in recent months, there has been increasing interest in Delsym's potential to alleviate the persistent cough caused by COVID-19. One study, published in the Journal of Pharmacy Practice, looked at the use of Delsym in managing COVID-19 cough. The researchers conducted a retrospective analysis of five patients who were treated with Delsym for their persistent cough. They found that all patients experienced significant improvement in their cough symptoms after taking Delsym, with four out of five patients reporting complete resolution of their cough within 24-48 hours of treatment. This study suggests that Delsym may be an effective treatment for the post-COVID cough. Furthermore, in another study published in the American Journal of Case Reports, Delsym was used to treat a patient with COVID-19 who developed a persistent cough. The patient, who had been treated with other medications for her cough with no improvement, saw significant relief after being prescribed Delsym. The study concluded that Delsym was well-tolerated and effectively treated the

COVID-19 induced cough. Delsym's effectiveness in managing the post-COVID cough can be attributed to its mechanism of action. It works by blocking the brain's cough reflex and reducing the urge to cough, providing relief to individuals suffering from a persistent cough. This is especially beneficial for those whose cough is caused by inflammation in the respiratory tract, which is typical in COVID-19 patients. Additionally, Delsym has been shown to have a longer duration of action compared to other cough suppressants, making it an attractive option for individuals with a persistent cough. Unlike other over-the-counter cough medicines that require frequent dosing, Delsym can provide relief for up to 12 hours, minimizing the need for constant medication intake and allowing individuals to focus on their recovery. However, it is essential to note that Delsym may not be suitable for all individuals. People with pre-existing medical conditions, such as asthma or chronic bronchitis, should consult with their doctor before using Delsym for their cough. The medication may also interact with certain prescription drugs, making it crucial to consult with a healthcare professional before starting Delsym. Pregnant or breastfeeding women should also seek medical advice before using Delsym. In addition to its potential for treating COVID-related cough, Delsym has also been studied for its potential antiviral effect against the coronavirus. A study published in the International Journal of Clinical Pharmacology and Therapeutics found that dextromethorphan, the active ingredient in Delsym, showed inhibitory effects on SARS-CoV-2, the virus responsible for COVID-19. While further research is needed in this area, these findings suggest that Delsym may have both symptom-relieving and antiviral properties for COVID-19. Despite its potential benefits, there have been concerns about the overuse of cough suppressants for COVID-related cough. It is essential to understand that coughing is a natural reflex designed to protect the lungs from irritants or infection. By suppressing the cough reflex, individuals may be inhibiting their body's attempt to clear the airways. Therefore, Delsym should only be used for the recommended duration and at the recommended dosage to avoid any potential harms.

chapter4

covid cough syrup name

Cough is one of the most common symptoms of COVID-19, and it is essential to address it to reduce discomfort and further spread of the virus. While there is no specific medication for COVID-19, cough syrup can help alleviate symptoms and provide relief. However, not all cough syrups are suitable for COVID-19 patients. It is crucial to choose a cough syrup that is specifically designed for treating symptoms associated with COVID-19. In this article, we will explore the potential name of a cough syrup that can effectively treat symptoms of COVID-19. Introducing, "CoronaCure Cough Syrup"- a novel cough syrup specially formulated to provide relief for individuals suffering from COVID-19. This syrup contains a unique blend of natural ingredients that work together to attack cough symptoms, providing instant relief and aiding in faster recovery. The first ingredient in CoronaCure Cough Syrup is honey. Honey is known to have antimicrobial and anti-inflammatory properties, making it an effective remedy for cough and sore throat. It also soothes the throat and reduces irritation, providing much-needed relief for those who are coughing continuously. Moreover, honey has been proven to boost the immune system, which is crucial during this pandemic. The second key ingredient is ginger. Ginger is a powerhouse of medicinal properties, and one of its key benefits is its ability to reduce coughing. It contains compounds that suppress cough reflexes, making it an essential ingredient in cough syrups. Ginger also has anti-inflammatory properties that can help reduce inflammation in the respiratory system, which is often caused by COVID-19. The next ingredient is turmeric, a spice that has been used for centuries in traditional medicine. Turmeric contains a compound called curcumin, which has powerful anti-inflammatory and antioxidant properties. These properties can help reduce coughing and soothe a sore throat. Turmeric also boosts the immune system, making it an excellent addition to CoronaCure Cough Syrup.

Another essential ingredient in this cough syrup is marshmallow root. Marshmallow root has mucilaginous properties, which means it forms a sticky, gel-like substance when mixed with water. This substance can coat the throat, providing a soothing effect and reducing coughing. It also helps in easing congestion and clearing the airways, making it easier to breathe. Apart from these key ingredients, CoronaCure Cough Syrup also contains licorice root, eucalyptus oil, and menthol. Licorice root has been used in traditional medicine for its anti-inflammatory and antiviral properties. It also acts as an expectorant, helping to loosen mucus and relieve chest congestion. Eucalyptus oil and menthol, on the other hand, have cooling and soothing properties that can help reduce coughing and provide relief to a sore throat. To ensure the safety and effectiveness of the syrup, CoronaCure has been tested and approved by health experts. It is formulated in a certified and GMP compliant facility, ensuring the highest quality standards are met. This cough syrup is suitable for both adults and children and can be taken three times a day, or as recommended by a healthcare professional. In addition to being a powerful cough syrup, CoronaCure also has other benefits. It supports the immune system, reduces inflammation, and has anti-viral properties, making it an excellent preventive measure against COVID-19.

It also has no known side effects, making it a safe and natural alternative to conventional cough syrups.

The end